I0414835

FOSS for Health Primer

FOSS for Health Primer

Dr. Nandalal Gunaratne

Dr. Pamela Patdu

and

Dr. Alvin B. Marcelo

Copyright © 2010 by Dr. Nandalal Gunaratne, Dr. Pamela Patdu, and Dr. Alvin B. Marcelo

ISBN: Softcover   978-1-4535-2085-7
               Ebook   978-1-4535-2086-4

All rights reserved. No part of this book may be reproduced or transmitted in any form
or by any means, electronic or mechanical, including photocopying, recording, or by
any information storage and retrieval system, without permission in writing from the
copyright owner.

This book was printed in the United States of America.

To order additional copies of this book, contact:
Xlibris Corporation
1-888-795-4274
www.Xlibris.com
Orders@Xlibris.com
71735

Contents

Introduction

Health

Health is defined by the World Health Organization as "a state of physical, mental and social well-being and not merely the absence of disease or infirmity."[1] It is essential to peace, security and happiness of all peoples and is viewed to be the ultimate aim of all economic and social development. [2]

Healthcare is recognized today as a global concern. Awareness of how health is affected by global trends in economy, politics, and environment supports this. For instance, with the growth of economies and development of technologies, it has become easier for people to move from country to country. People then become susceptible to diseases in the destination country which was previously unknown or rare in their native land. Also, migration becomes a means by which an unknown or rare disease is carried into a recipient country. Even the movement of goods like food can carry diseases.

Environmental pollution has contributed to increasing respiratory morbidity and mortality. Global warming has been correlated with an increase in cardiovascular morbidity and mortality and even increases in diseases like malaria and dengue. Natural disasters like volcanic eruptions, floods, and hurricanes have been affecting people in many countries. The recent Indian Ocean Tsunami was an extreme example. These such disasters impact the health scenario by increasing mortality and the demands for rehabilitation. Also, these decrease food supply because of the destruction of crops and farms, and subsequently add to the burden of malnutrition.

Indeed, health is a shared responsibility. Governments around the world have endeavored to improve their healthcare delivery systems consistent with the WHO principle that "the attainment of the highest standard of health is the fundamental right of every human being without distinction of race, religion, political belief, economic or social condition." [3] Today, problems and criticisms on health systems in both developed and developing nations continue to exist and is not confined to just anyone of these domains of healthcare:

1. Primary care—the first place of encounter at the community level
2. Secondary care—level at which primary care physicians refer to
3. Tertiary care—is specialist care in a specialist hospital setting with facilities

In all these three domains, the health issues can be summarized into these[4][5][6][7] :

1. equity
2. accessibility
3. affordability
4. availability
5. quality
6. appropriateness

Strategies in addressing these issues in health can be encapsulated in the WHO agenda which is based on six points, that in turn address two health objectives, two strategic needs, and two operational approaches:[8]

1. Promoting Development
2. Fostering Health Security
3. Strengthening Health Systems
4. Harnessing Research, Information and Evidence
5. Enhancing Partnerships
6. Improving Performance

Health Informatics

Industries and government agencies have adopted Information and Communication Technology (ICT) successfully. Industries like the banking industry and share brokering, have shown what a great difference it makes. Multi-nationals have also used ICT very successfully to run their transnational business far more efficiently than before.

Healthcare is an industry that can also potentially benefit vastly from the adoption of ICT as it is an information-intensive industry. This is reaffirmed by the WHO agenda of "harnessing research, information and evidence"[9] To be able to deliver a high standard of healthcare, it needs to have interoperability between different healthcare institutions, to keep up-to-date health statistics and ever-growing research, manage stores, medical records, images, and drugs, and plan delivery geared to particular needs. The use of paper-based information creates a huge mass of illegible data that is susceptible to loss. The data has to be manually analyzed, and this takes such a long time, that in many countries the analyzed health data lags behind a few years. Keeping the enormous amounts of paper that needs space and protection from elements like animals and fungi. Adopting ICT then seems to be a good idea.

In fact, notions of health informatics—the acquisition, storage, retrieval and use of information for healthcare—has dated back to the 1950's when terms like medical computing, medical information processing, computer medicine and medical software engineering have already been used.[10] There has also been formal government support since the 1960's. The Agency for healthcare Research and Quality (AHRQ) and its predecessors, for example, has had a more than 30-year history of support for medical informatics projects broadly divided into medical information systems, decision support and quality assurance and computer-based medical records.[11]

Benefits from medical informatics have presently been shown to deal with present health issues that span accessibility, availability, cost, and quality.

Why is the healthcare industry slow in adopting ICT?

Despite the fact that the value of digitized information to the healthcare industry is accepted by many governments, the actual adoption of ICT has been slow. The possible reasons are:

1. There has been few successful implementations to show the cost-benefit in broad terms.
2. The cost of implementation is high, both for hardware/communication as well as for software.
3. A lack of expertise and ICT literacy by the domain experts
4. Inconsistencies in the industry and failure of support to live up to the standards expected. Failure of interoperability between applications even by the same software producer!
5. A lack of priority by many governments to the use of ICT in healthcare.

This primer discusses the potential of Free/Open Source Software, open standards and open content in maximizing ICT to address present health issues and contribute in improving the standards of healthcare.

What is FOSS?

When software was first written years ago, in the days of the early unix kernal, the source code was available for all to see, to try out changes, to modify to their needs and to exchange with friends and colleagues. As the ICT industry developed, this changed. Companies claimed ownership of software via copyrights and patents in view of protecting their profits and investments. Most of the widely-used software on desktops have then belonged to proprietary companies. The source code, which is copyrighted to the company, was made unavailable for others to study, modify and improve in collaboration. Such software is now termed "closed source software."

Disturbed by this turn of events, some people in the software industry, including Richard Stallmann, started the free software movement to bring freedom in software development and promote the sharing of knowledge. These software had a concept of "copyleft", the antithesis of copyright, which restricts users to the use and modification of software if only these modifications will also be released with a similar license. Different licenses under "copyleft" like the GNU General Public License and the GNU Lesser General Public license illustrate the concept of Free and Open Source Systems and defends four freedoms that the Free Software Foundation defines:

- Freedom to run a program for any purpose
- Freedom to study the program and adopt it to the person's needs
- The freedom to make and redistribute copies to anyone you like
- Give the improvements you did to the program back to the community

The Internet gave these groups a free environment to grow, and the Free (for freedom) Open Source Software movement began to grow and grow.

From the start, FOSS did allow people the freedom to sell the software and also support the software for a fee. This made it possible for people to make a living out of FOSS, and FOSS-based business opportunities started to develop.

The FOSS model became a basis for commercial and community integration and collaboration, each recognizing the value of the other. Some of these commercial companies became well-known, like RedHat. Major players like Netscape started to involve themselves with the FOSS movement and community, bringing in a lot of their closed code and making it open. This resulted in some very useful software coming into the field and increasing the number of quality FOSS. Today, majority of web servers are run under the FOSS platform. Examples of software already at the forefront are:

1. Open Office which follows the open document protocols was from source provided by Sun Microsystems.
2. Mozilla Project which includes the Firefox web browser, was from source provided by the Netscape browser project.
3. Java and a host of Java based software like the Tomcat web server from Sun Microsystems.

As these core software gain ground in the market of IT, FOSS' popularity has extended to revolutionizing different fields like education and government service. In the following section, we will explore how FOSS can impact healthcare.

FOSS in healthcare

FOSS has powerful, well-built, widely-used software architectures that form the basis of many FOSS healthcare software. The LAMP[12] stack is the best known. Linux[13]—the Operating System, Apache[14]—the web browser, MySQL[15] or PostgreSQL[16] the RDMS and PHP[17]/Python[18]/PERL,[19] the scripting languages, form LAMP. The Java[20]-based version of this uses Jakarta Tomcat[21] instead of Apache and Java instead of the other listed languages. Another popular platform is ZOPE[22] (Z Objects Presentation Environment) which is a python-based web application server. Though these work best in the Unix/Linux environment, these softwares are truly cross-platform, working in MS Windows and MacOSX.

Most healthcare software built on FOSS make use of the above software. The question is, what is it about FOSS that makes it a good platform in which to adopt ICT in healthcare? The answer lies in similarity in both foundations of principle and practice.

We must note that the four freedoms that open source software defends give rise to a unique development method that distinguishes it from closed source software. It provides:

1. Reduced cost of maintenance due to costs being shared by the users, who add code and fix bugs, and the organization, which maintains the software, makes enhancements and provides support. Also, cost is reduced as there is no need to pay for licensing and other proprietary fees.
2. The reduction of effort duplication as people are able to build on the work of others across the world and the preservation of all these efforts. There is no more danger of losing present developments as proprietary vendors' business goes out of the market and leave their closed system unmaintained and unadaptable to present the needs of an institution or organization.
3. The ability to change very fast with regard improvements, bug fixing, and adaptations, resulting in better quality control, way beyond what is possible with conventional software. Since lower costs attract more users, more users are able to test the software and report problems. Furthermore, the above platforms are all well-known, tried and tested applications and there are many programmers and users who are familiar with them potentially producing a larger pool of people who can fix bugs in the applications. This, in part, addresses the barrier of a lack of know-how to deal with IT seen in proprietary systems—the procurement, and subsequently the study of which, are constrained by costs and license limitations. Also, FOSS often comes hand in hand with a version system, that allows for multiple users to make improvements without fear of damaging what has already been done. These such improvements are then again available for deployment in the public and quality control can go on.
4. Better adherence to open standards facilitated by its accessibility and its projected large user base. FOSS' popularity and inherent accessibility ensure a common ground on which to build on interoperability and use of standards for data transfer across applications. Such common ground is difficult to reach in the presence of closed source codes.

In summary, the above method provides advantages in addressing cost reduction, availability, accessibility, efficiency, and quality in the use of ICT in health, very much akin to answering the present challenges of healthcare, as previously discussed. In principle, addressing these issues boil down to working towards making the highest standard of health truly a fundamental right of everyone. Furthermore, the whole notion of collaboration, as propagated by the Open Source Movement is at home to the principle that health is a shared responsibility and to the foundations of the scientific method which promotes sharing of information and peer review to contribute to the growth of knowledge.

Indeed, the potentials of Free/Open Source Software in health care are evident. However, as much as success has been met in other industries, FOSS in health should address the aspects that make health care different.

A survey of current FOSS

Free/Open source software have been used in the clinics, hospital and community setting. This section will introduce the areas where FOSS have been used in health care: Clinical Practice Management, Hospital Management and Information Systems, Personal Health Records, Decision Support and Quality Assurance, Public Health, and Medical Research.

Clinical Practice Management

This is software used by clinicians to take care of day-to-day operations of their practice including facilitating billing and recording patient demographics, scheduled appointments, and progress notes.

Hospital Management and Information Systems

This is a more comprehensive software for the administration and management of a hospital. Some are suitable for small rural hospitals while others are usable in the large, complex hospitals. This software has to look after the many areas like radiology, nuclear medicine, surgical stores, staff management, payment to staff, laboratory, pathology, out-patients and in-patient care, radiotherapy, physiotherapy and many other units that maybe found in a hospital.

The modules common to all of them include:

1. A patient registry—is a system to gather clinical and other data to achieve particular objectives like quality service assurance, description of natural history of a disease and epidemiology.

2. Electronic Medical Record—is a system that provides real time access to data concerning medical care. Handling of data must involve proper authentication and must adhere to access, privacy, and confidentiality policies.
3. Scheduling—aids in allocation of appointments.
4. Billing—facilitates bill issuance, collections reporting, and payment status.
5. Insurance—is involved in claim facilitation, automatic payments, and accounting of insurance payments
6. Pharmacy—facilitates recording and reporting of refill compliance, inventory control and prescription writing

Personal Health Records

The concept of personal health records maintained and owned by citizens, has been promoted increasingly with the spread of the Internet and the increasing ICT literacy of the population in general.

One of the most important issues that will have to be considered are patient identification. In a forum conducted by the National Alliance for Health Information Technology—NAHIT, entitled "Identification of Patients: A Technical and Cultural Challenge That Can No Longer Be Avoided,[23]" consisted of a panel session of experts and facilitated breakout sessions, which revealed a number of common themes-

- Regional versus national: There is significant debate of whether the responsibility for matching patients with their records lies at the regional or the national level. The group articulated benefits of both models.
- Value proposition: The value proposition for a national network of connected health records must be more fully articulated for all involved stakeholders.
- Consumer/patient: Consumers must first be engaged and educated on the value of health IT in order for them to fully trust it and embrace its use.
- Policy: Further discussion must take place at the policy level in order to clarify the unique needs brought by health information technology. Terminology in these conversations must correlate with consumer engagement efforts to avoid confusion for all those involved.

- Technology: There are similar terminology disconnects regarding the technology of matching patients with their records, and these must be resolved. Although there are significant differences between the two most often discussed technological methods of matching, commonalities exist that will provide the seeds of consensus.

The advantages of citizens having their own records include:

Independence and responsibility for them, including security and decisions of what is available for them, what they will share and what they will not. They will also be partly responsible for the security of their data.

The availability independent of geographical boundaries.

Improve the knowledge of the citizen as he keeps the record updated and accurate as possible.

Decision Support and Quality Assurance

These are systems that aim to gather data for the purposes of producing point-of-care recommendations that improve the quality of care of physicians.

Public Health

These include applications that deal with acquisition, storage and reporting of data for the purposes of public health. As a public health tool, it emphasizes on data that deals more with populations rather than individuals. It often involves a range of tools like report generation and reporting systems, business intelligence tools, geographic information systems, statistical analysis software

Medical Research

Medical research applications are able to facilitate clinical studies by providing tools for data submission, validation, filtering and extraction. It also allows for reporting and oversight of the studies. The leading open source clinical research application is OpenClinica. It has an LGPL open source license and is commercially supported by Akaza Research which has been created with the goal of promoting shared tools, repositories, and open standards for public research.[24]

Some other applications in medical research facilitate search for online medical literature. An example of this is BioMail.[25]

Look at the appendix for more examples.

Medical Imaging

Medical imaging applications includes image creation, acquisition, storage, management and distribution of medical images. More capabilities for extraction, merging and transformation of medical content from several images are now being developed. [26]

For a comprehensive list of FOSS, see the appendix.

FOSS in Asia-Pacific

The Free/Open Source Software movement has extended to include

Patient Registry: ISIS

ISIS is a system used by the Department of Surgery, Philippine General Hospital (PGH). It is a software application that has been built on the LAMP architecture presently running in the intranet of the PGH. It has been started in 2004 when a grant was given by the Foundation for the Advancement of Surgical Education (FASE). It is presently the largest patient registry in the Philippines containing more than a hundred thousand records and has been referenced in several publications. Generation of official insurance forms, clinical abstracts and discharge summaries are accomplished by ISIS.

PCDOM Primacare

PrimaCare is an open source electronic health records and clinical management system born in a setting where typical clinics do not have access to expensive proprietary health information systems due to the prohibitive costs of licenses. It presently has modules on system administration, clinic management, financial management, patient management, prescription, billing, schedule, asset and supplies management and medical resources. It is looking into the development of a Generic Engine for Modules (GEM) software to aid in developing modules by providing databases, business logics, user interfaces, and report templates.

Hospital Information Systems: Hospital OS in Thailand

Hospital OS[27] is Thailand's first open-source hospital information system in Thailand. It is financially supported by the Thailand Research Fund and it is available at no cost for those who have chosen to use it as in the 50 hospitals in Thailand at present. This information system is a cross-platform solution in Java running a PostgreSQL database developed by a team of programmers, software engineers, health professionals and hospital experts. It is designed to facilitate efficient data reporting, filing and processing in the hospital and includes modules on Registration, Medical Records, Patient Screening Counter, X-Ray, Laboratory, Pharmacy, Medical Statistic, and in-patient department cashier.

The Hospital OS's IT system consultants provide on-site voluntary support and coordination with the different hospitals in terms of user training, software implementation and software customization according to a particular hospital's needs. A web board is another means by which the government units and end users in the community hospitals collaborate to provide inputs in the development of Hospital OS, report bugs, and share experiences and best practices in working with the system. The sharing of best practices aims to make the use of Hospital OS sustainable by making knowhow of the system as a resource that is preserved, continually expanded and shared by the users. Being an open source software then presents advantages to easily integrate these best practices into the work flow of the system. Furthermore, as these community hospitals in Thailand are seen as centers of local community development, the online collaboration provided by the system aims to involve a wider grassroots level of knowledge sharing and development that can hopefully be propagated on a national scale.

Hospital Information Systems: VistA in Pakistan

The Shaukat Khanum Memorial Center Hospital and Research Center (SKMCH-RC) in Pakistan is a cancer and research center that was aided by the US State Department to run VistA in their hospital by giving financial support, maintenance, capacity development of SKM professionals

Bajwa identifies the reasons why the use of VistA did not take off in this hospital. [28]

1. There was a perceived lack of strategy in the local adoption of the system. Only 2 out of the 27 departments made use of the system.
2. There was lack of sustainable expertise. The two people who were trained in the US to handle the VistA system in SKMHC, left Pakistan after 4 months in SKMCH-RC because they were hired by hospitals using VistA in the US. Their knowhow was not passed on to anybody so nobody was able to add subsequent modules for the other remaining systems in the hospital that are in need of the information system.
3. At the time of adoption, there was also dissatisfaction because of the lack of graphical user interface and the complexity of having several screen interfaces to do a simple task.

Bajwa suggests that the project could have been a success if[29]

1. End-user involvement was encouraged
2. There are dedicated personnel to handle upgrade management
3. Communities of learning and practice were encouraged
4. There were established support and management teams and organizations
5. There was communication with the larger user community

Hospital Information Systems: VistA in the National Cancer Institute and Nasser Institute Hospital, Egypt

VistA was first adopted in Egypt in 1990 in the form of its predecessor, the Decentralized Hospital Computer Program (DHCP), by the National Cancer Institute-Cairo University. The software was then built on MUMPS and was not formally an open source application. However, the Veteran's Affairs who owned VistA, allowed for its source code to be modified according to the hospitals like NCI that choose to deploy it. Programs that were used include Patient Registration, Inpatient Admissions/ Discharges/ Transfers (ADT), Surgery, Laboratory, Pharmacy, Radiology, Record Tracking, Nursing, Engineering, and a test version of the Clinical Imaging module. [30] In-house developed applications like Radiotherapy,

Histopathology, Cytopathology and Osteomies are also run alongside these core VistA modules.

Several issues needed to be addressed in the deployment of VistA in the National Cancer Institute. First, there were no programmers available to work with VistA and Mumps. A team was trained by flying in experts from the US and Germany. Some of the programmers were also sent to the US for training. Second, there was a need for localization of VistA. While medical education in Egypt was done in English, other projected users in the hospital could only understand and work with Arabic. Also, for accuracy, names of patient and staff had to be in Arabic. Together with the customization for the hospital's needs, Arabization was done in-house with some help from the staff of Veteran Affairs staff and University of Wurzburg, Germany.

Another issue was that a lot of the end users are not used to using computers. There was then a 2-step training for the staff. The first step was basic computer use such as typing practice, printing, and even turning the computer on and off. The second step consisted of training on using VistA itself. Trainers designated were as much as possible coming from the same field as the trainee. For instance, nurses trained nurses and internists trained other internists.

Another roadblock was the establishment of support for the project. Initially, experts from the US assisted in the initial setup of the applications. Formal relationships on a management level was established with Veteran Affairs. Also, online communications and support was provided by the Washington ISC, Silver Spring. Dr. Omar Al Attab, who led the implementation of VistA in NCI, cites that the presence of many international experts from whom they can ask support from helped a lot in making VistA work for them. Internal support was also strong from the deans and the hospital administrators.

At present, the NCI continues to use VistA after two major hardware upgrades and a software upgrade. Data from 1992 are still accessible and are utilized in patient's day to day care and also in research and cancer registration. It was noted that the use of Common Procedure Terminology(CPT) codes and International Code for Diseases (ICD) and SNOMED in VistA was viewed as very helpful in facilitating research. [31]

The success of VistA in NCI has already attracted many to adopt VistA. In 1997, the Hospital Management Information Systems (HIMS) Project was started in Egypt and was supported by the Egyptian Government and the USAID. It aimed to establish a hospital information system in the 4 hospitals and headquarters of the Cairo Curative Organization-Ministry of

Health and Population. In 1999, the Nasser Hospital Institute joined this project. The deployment was aided by Maximus[32], an organization that serves as an enabler of governments, one of the services provided by which is systems development, integration and implementation services to public health sector services. Maximus provided the training for programmers, system administrators, troubleshooters and hardware support staff. Each task performed by Maximus had a counterpart point person among the Egyptian staff who will perform these same jobs when Maximus is gone. For each module in VistA that will be utilized in NIH, Maximus trained a member of the HMIS department and a staff of the department concerned with the module. These people are then tasked to teach what they have learned to their respective departments. Maximus also set up a computer lab for training of 300 employees on basic computer skills. This new skills encouraged the staff to participate in the project. All throughout the process of deployment, feedback from the end users were used in the catering the VistA modules to the needs of the hospital. Within a year, training of hospital staff and network infrastructure installation was accomplished.

Public Health: CHITS (http://chits.mudfish.info/ | http://developer.berlios.de/projects/chits/)

The Philippine health information systems, in literature, has been characterized by the presence of high levels of duplication and delays due to manual processing. In addition, no quality control on the data from paper forms exist and no means of feedback are given back to the collectors of the data and the community. There was no systematic method of storing collected data to make it easily retrievable for analysis and decision-making. With the trends of emigration of doctors from the communities, the information systems are also left to be managed by local health workers. In this setting, Community Health Information Tracking System (CHITS) was started as a collaboration between the University of the Philippines Medical Informatics Unit and the University of Philippines College of Medicine Section of Community Medicine in 2004. Initial funding of CHITS was granted by PANASIA-ICT. The CHITS was designed to address the information management issues at the level of the local health center, making it capable of integrating with information systems at the higher municipal level. The bigger picture was that this move to improve local health information infrastructure was seen as a step towards the vision of building a national health infrastructure in five years.

On the ground, what CHITS had to deal with are the limited access to technology and funding and the lack of knowhow of local community workers in handling information systems such as CHITS.

These problems were addressed on several fronts. Technically, the system was designed with an open source modular architecture. The open source approach reduced costs as opposed to using proprietary software and also promotes the transparency in how the data, which is valuable to the community, is processed. The modular architecture contributed to the scalability of the project so that immediate needs can be prioritized over others in a setting of limited time and technical resources. For instance, in the earlier phases of the project the development of the clinical module was prioritized over modules for the vertical programs which the local health workers needed most to generate the reports required of them. Also, this modularity facilitated the involvement of the local health workers in the development of their CHITS interface from picking colors to deciding what data fields they need. Their role as owners of their CHITS are then emphasized with this level of involvement to increase the incentive for them to support the system and ensure its sustainability.

Integration of capacity building of the local community workers was done with the deployment of CHITS. These locals were taught skills starting from the basics like opening the computer and using the mouse by utilizing fun strategies like making them play games first. Later on, they were then exposed to the CHITS interface. Later on, those local workers who have gained the skills are then expected to teach new workers that join them. This process is formalized into a certification course on data management to emphasize the importance of keeping data accurate and valid among the local health workers.

Internal and external resources were also tapped for funding and further support. Stakeholders of the vertical programs like the implementing arm of the WHO Directly Observed Therapy for Shortcourse, The Philippine Coalition against Tuberculosis (PhilCAT), has been enjoined to support the sustainability of the project. With the success met in the pilot areas, collaboration with other local government units, who are in turn able to find other internal and external sources of support, are now being done. [33]

Humanitarian: SAHANA

The Sahana Disaster Management System's primary objective is to help alleviate human suffering and save lives through the efficient use of IT. It purports to address coordination problems like finding missing people, managing aid, managing volunteers, providing disaster situation updates, tracking camps and needs effectively between groups, non-governmental organizations and victims.

Its development was started by ICT volunteers in Sri Lanka and supported by the Lanka Software Foundation as a response to the needs of helping out the families and communities devastated by the Indian Ocean Tsunami in year 2004. At this time, hundreds of thousands of people were affected and infrastructure was destroyed. After three weeks of development of Sahana, it was initially deployed in 2004 by the Sri Lankan government's Center of National Operations to track victims and coordinate volunteers.

After the Tsunami, Sahana was rebuilt from scratch on the LAMP (Linux, Apache, MySQL, PHP) architecture to be a free, open source software itself. This was done because, an open source system was seen to address the demands of the disaster situations in terms of an open approach, cost reduction, and adaptability.[34]

A lot of humanitarian groups believe in transparency and grassroots involvement as in the approach of the open source movement which makes the system globally-owned and open to the development of anyone. Such transparency was deemed important to promote trust in the collaboration of various stakeholders like nongovernmental organizations and government institutions among them.

It has been noted that a lot of response in disaster situations are weakened due to a lack of funding. In both developed and developing nations, such lack of funding springs from the lack of impetus to support something which may or may not happen. Cost reduction from savings on licensing costs and shared global development then further supported the use of an open source platform.

The need for adaptability, akin to disaster situations which are often sporadic events happening in different areas, also well fit the open source paradigm because the availability of code made it easy for developers to cater the system according to particular local needs

Sahana has been designed to cater to the needs of security and scalability. Sahana has provisions for authentication mechanisms on changes made to the system by the different groups involved for security. Furthermore, it is very scalable since its designed to be deployed on a single computer without networking capabilities or it can be extended to a wide area network of computers depending on resources available. Also, it has a modular design where components can be plugged in or out depending on the needs of the situation.

Later on, the development team has been coordinating with various groups to promote the free/open source Sahana to be able to extend its use in other disasters. It has already been used to respond to

1. the AsianQuake in Pakistan in 2005 as deployed by National Database Registration Authority (NADRA) and the Government of Pakistan with the support of IBM country teams
2. the Southern Leyte Mudslide Disaster in the Philippines in 2006 as deployed by the National Disaster Coordinating Council (NDCC) and Philippine Office of Civil Defense (OCD) for the Philippine Government with the support of IBM country teams
3. the Sarvodaya in Sri Lanka in 2006 as deployed by Sri Lanka's largest NGO
4. the Terre des Hommes in Sri Lanka in 2006
5. the Yogjarkata Earthquake in Indonesia in 2006 as deployed by urRemote, Indonesian Whitewater Association and Indian Rescue Source, sponspored by Australian Computer Society

The Sahana Disaster Management System has six full time developers. It is supported by the Lanka Software Foundation(LSF), a non-profit foundation that promotes FOSS among Sri Lankan developers. Aside from the full time developers, there have been a lot of people involved in the Sahana Community including over a hundred disaster management experts, emergency management practitioners, humanitarian consultants, nongovernmental organizations, academics, and FOSS developers from Sri Lanka, United Kingdom, United States, New Zealand, Australia, Thailand and other parts of the world.

The biggest challenges that the LSF faces today is to continue to have financial support from commercial companies, aid agencies, universities and individuals.[35]

Sources of information about FOSS

As advocates of FOSS in healthcare increase, updates in the developments around the world are very important. The Open Source Health Care Alliance (OSHCA) is a non-profit organization that aims to promote FOSS.

It provides a comprehensive list of FOSS at http://oshca.org/healthdir/fosshealthapps.

Other sources of information about FOSS are:

- Journal of Open Source Medical Computing (http://www.josmc.org)
- OpenClinical.Org (http://www.openclinical.org/)
- Wikipedia (http://en.wikipedia.org/wiki/List_of_open_source_healthcare)
- LinuxMedNews(http://linuxmednews.com)
- *NewsForge Medical (http://newsforge.com/search.pl?query=medical)*
- US: The Open Source Reference Book (http://www.egovos.org/Resources/Book)
- EMRUPDATE (http://emrupdate.com)
- *GPL Medicine (http://gplmedicine.org)*
- *Inventory of Evaluation Studies of health Informatics (http://evaldb.umit.at)*

Open Standards

Standards in technical usage is a framework of specifications that has been:

- approved by a recognized organization, or
- is generally accepted and widely used throughout the industry.

A related concept is that of interoperability. It must be noted that standards and interoperability are not the same thing. Standards are much narrower and specify technical details. Interoperability, on the other hand, is a much broader concept that involves both a technical and business context. Interoperability is defined as the ability of different information technology systems and software applications to communicate, to exchange data accurately, effectively, and consistently, and to use the information that has been exchanged. [36]

Standards and provisions for interoperability ensure that products and services are of adequate quality and that they work together even though they maybe from different parties and entities. Ultimately they raise the quality, safety, reliability, efficiency and interoperability, and provide such benefits at an economical cost. [15]

In the IT industry, for example, ISO/IEC 9126 is a standard that provides a framework for the evaluation of software quality. It does not provide requirements for softwares, but it defines a quality model which is applicable to every kind of software. In particular, it defines six product quality characteristics: [37]

1. functionality
2. usability
3. maintability
4. reliability
5. efficiency
6. portablity

In an annex, this standard also provides a suggestion of quality sub characteristics.

Why standards are important in healthcare

Health standards are important to maintain high quality of services in the health profession as these services highly impact the quality of life of people. There is also an increasing imperative for the health care services to be able to interact with each other. This need is heightened by the increasing mobility of people that results in increasing the number of health institutions they go to. As such, as they move about from one provider to another there is a need for these providers to interact and pass on health data to ensure the continuity of care of these people. Also, as more and more people, organizations and businesses are now involved in health care systems development and more and more systems are deployed at the different levels of healthcare around the world. How old and new healthcare players interact then becomes a greater challenge. The accuracy of the transmission of data on diagnoses, epidemiological data, drug regimes of a patient and its subsequent readability and usability through the different systems that underlie technologies are needed to deliver quality care to patients. Various studies have shown that errors in these areas account for unnecessary morbidity and mortality[38] and that these can be reduced by the use of effective health IT[39] [40] [41]. Today, moves towards the assurance of quality and communication among these systems are made possible with the establishment of standards and provisions of interoperability.

How do health standards develop?

Standards develop in one of three ways. One is dictated by the market (e.g.: pdf file system) called *de facto,* and the other by consensus by many people in a large SDO (HL 7 messaging standard) called *de jure* and lastly, industry-driven, where some industrial group creates and formalizes a standard (e.g.: Open Document Standard).

Standards are set by Standard-Setting Organizations (SSO), like the International Organization for Standardization (ISO) and the International Telecommunication Union (ITU).

How do SDOs develop a health standard?

In the U.S., many of these organizations are accredited by the American National Standards Institute (ANSI), under which the development process must fulfill four main requirements[42]:

Openness—*any parties in the United States directly influenced by the activity can participate in the development process.*

Balance—*the task forces developing the standards are composed of a balanced distribution of stakeholder groups in order to ensure that no single group can influence the development of a standard to favor their own interests.*

Consensus—*substantial agreement has been reached by directly and materially affected interest categories. In addition to a majority opinion being required for a standard to pass ballot, all views and objections must be considered and an effort made toward their resolution.*

Due process—*this provides for broad-based public review and comment on draft standards, and includes an appeals process for any who feel this process was not met.*

In the USA, under the initiatives of the President of the country[43], a decision was made to adopt common standards for Healthcare ICT. Since the USA is a leading player in software development as well as standards development, these standards are likely to be adopted by most countries. Indeed there is already collaboration across countries in testing and developing these standards.

The reasons given in this US based initiative for the importance of interoperability in developing policy, were as follows[17] :

Policy:

In fulfilling its responsibilities, the work of the National Coordinator shall be consistent with a vision of developing a nationwide interoperable health information technology infrastructure that:

(a) *Ensures that appropriate information to guide medical decisions is available at the time and place of care;*
(b) *Improves healthcare quality, reduces medical errors, and advances the delivery of appropriate, evidence-based medical care;*
(c) *Reduces healthcare costs resulting from inefficiency, medical errors, inappropriate care, and incomplete information;*
(d) *Promotes a more effective marketplace, greater competition, and increased choice through the wider availability of accurate information on healthcare costs, quality, and outcomes;*
(e) *Improves the coordination of care and information among hospitals, laboratories, physician offices, and other ambulatory care providers through an effective infrastructure for the secure and authorized exchange of healthcare information; and*
(f) *Ensures that patients' individually identifiable health information is secure and protected.*

Open standards defined

There are several standards that have been developed in healthcare but they have not been uniformly implemented even in the same country. There have been instances where the new version of a standard has been incompatible with the previous version.

The problem has become that, healthcare has too many standards in some areas (messaging, language) and none in others (allergies). Many competing standards are as bad as no standards, as they result in failure of different HIT software to speak to each other. Therefore industry-led open standards developed by SDOs with international collaboration, seems the only reliable way forward. Open standards will be of greater benefit to all as they are not tied to a particular vendor or a country. The value of FOSS for the implementation of such standards become apparent, as they will readily adopt these standards to remain compatible. Open standards are defined and described in another Primer. Generally, they have the following characteristics:

- easy accessibility for all to read and use;
- developed by a process that is open and relatively easy for anyone to participate in; and
- no control or tie-in by any specific group or vendor.

How open source software leverages the implementation of open standards and interoperability

Standards are meant to be used by players of the field consistently. For this to be possible, it needs adequate documentation and specification that are available to the public so that any potential player will be able to access it. Open source software may serve as an avenue to maintain reference implementation of standards set by Standards Development Organizations. The open source software components can then be used by developers or integrators to reduce costs of developments in implementations to be able to adopt to standards. The presence of a open source reference implementation also makes it possible to have an inclusive community involved to share their best practices and to test, validate and develop the standard through the reference implementation. Sfakianakis describes OpenECG and DICOM as standards that had reference implementations aid in the standards' acceptance and development. [44]

A Survey of Open Standards

Common domains of standards include terminology, data exchange or messaging, document standards, conceptual standards and architecture standards.[45]

An example of data exchange or messaging open standard is established by organizations like the Health Level Seven (HL7). This standard is widely-used in the United States and has now expanded to standards in terminology and decision support. This organization has also created a document standard, the Clinical Document Architecture.

There are also open standards for data acquisition, exchange, submission, and archiving for research like that established by the Clinical Data Interchange Standards Consortium.

Open Access and Open Content

Open content in healthcare

The definition for content that is used in the Open Content License is that[46]: "Content is just about anything that isn't executable". It could be anything digital—that is, anything that could be distributed or accessed electronically—that is not software. This sort of content could be images, audio files, movies and text.

Open content, coined by Dr. David Wiley in 1998 by analogy with "open source," describes any kind of creative work (including articles, pictures, audio, and video) or engineering work (i.e. open machine design) that is published in a format that explicitly allows the copying and the modifying of the information by anyone; not exclusively by a closed organization, firm or individual[47]. Content can be either in the public domain or under an open license like one of the Creative Commons Licenses[48]. The Creative Commons Licenses offers a range of possible restrictions while maintaining the notion of sharing of content, and these include:

1. Attribution—allows commercial and noncommercial use, redistribution and tweaking as long as there is acknowledgment accorded the sources
2. Share-alike—allows commercial and noncommercial use, redistribution and tweaking, as long as there is acknowledgment accorded the sources and the derivative works also have a share-alike license
3. No derivatives—for commercial and noncommercial use without modifying the original work, requires acknowledgment of source
4. Noncommercial—commercial use not allowed, can redistribute and tweak as long as there is acknowledgment of the source
5. Noncommercial Share Alike—commercial use not allowed, can redistribute and tweak as long as there is acknowledgment of the source

Well known Open Content Projects are: Wikipedia the on-line Free Encyclopedia[49] and the Open Directory Project[50].

Open Access[51] is a more restricted way of usage. In this context, OA means that an article is still protected by copyright but is distributed under a Creative Commons or similar license that generally allows more liberal use than a traditional copyrighted work. The license terms are not identical for all OA articles. License statements in each article stipulate specific terms of use.

Why is open content important in healthcare

Healthcare is an information intensive, knowledge based field. Continuous research throughout centuries have created wonders in what can be done in medicine. This research must not stop and must build on, challenge and expand what is already medical knowledge. Furthermore, easy access to this up-to-date knowledge on diseases, treatment, and processes can serve to be improve the delivery of care and thus, the quality of life of patients. Unfortunately, most healthcare publications and books that are needed by the domain specialist are becoming increasingly expensive. This is partly because it is being produced for a small niche market in small numbers.

This has created a divide between those who can afford to purchase these publications and those who cannot. The use of digital media across the Internet has made many of these publications available in the digital form, but the costs have not changed to benefit consumers.

The obvious result is the creation of a digital divide, with unequal distribution of knowledge with resulting loss of professional development as well as healthcare development in affected regions.

The development of Open Content related to healthcare has changed this considerably. Well-known Peer Reviewed Journals are now available for free reading, with or without restrictions. Some journals only allow free access to those journals older than a certain defined period e.g.: that are over 6 months old, or offer only abstracts, the full article has to be paid for.

Even with these limitations, the availability has created a better knowledge distribution in the healthcare domain.

How can we improve/increase access to more open content?

Open Content is seen as nihilistic by some academics. There are many criticisms of Open Content. It is mostly a development of the Internet. The content is added by many people. There may not be Peer Review, and the quality of the content maybe doubtful.

There are restrictions on the already published material, which maybe under copyrights. This may mean that they cannot be made available as open content, indeed, even if the original author, the creator of the content, may wish to do so. This is because these materials now belong to the publisher, and not the author, by previous agreement.

The whole idea of allowing the creation of someone, to be used by others, is anathema to the industry that has developed over the years on the bedrock of copyright laws. This gives ownership, a sense of security and belonging to the author of the material as well as the owner of the material. This may or not be the original author.

Collaboration and knowledge sharing has taken a new look in the Internet, remotely different to what was there before. The ease of access to not only content but to each other, has given rise to the sharing of information, solving problems and giving things away that has open new vistas in cooperative consumption. Wikipedia has shown how many inputs from a vast majority can create knowledge that is as good as that produced by a few expert authors over several years, costing much more in time, money and resources. The multi-lingual/multi-national/multi-cultural input makes the final result, richer.

Indeed, the popularity of open content and the awareness of the disparity in access to knowledge due to economic factors, has made its mark. Many health journals, books and other publications including multi-media content are being made available by traditionally "cagey" publishers. This is an acknowledgment that such availability adds to the popularity of the journal. Indeed, eventually, the number of people who read the journal, decides the success of the journal. More people will also publish in it. The growth of Open Content then relies today on having awareness of the availability of these resources and giving encouragement to use these to as many people as possible.

The Challenges Ahead: FOSS in 21st century healthcare

Healthcare presents continuing challenges and its importance as a shared responsibility cannot be denied in this age of ever-increasing movement of people around the world and of ever-expanding reach of technology. Decades of health informatics developments in the fields of clinic/hospital information management systems, decision support systems, public health, imaging, and research have been shown to contribute to improve the standards of care. The benefits of these health informatics ventures are not without detriments, however. The costs of acquiring health IT infrastructure has become prohibitive for some and thus serves to increase the inequity in health care. The increasing number of players in the field has presented problems with the communication among the health care providers. The demise of health IT companies left behind their locked old, irrelevant systems to the health providers.

In this primer, we have presented the paradigms of open source software, open standards and interoperability, and open content and access as applied to health to be viable working options that take advantage of the inherent strengths of information technology while being a cure to the ails that IT has previously brought forward. Open source software provide a vast array of applications in the different areas of healthcare. Open standards ensure the quality of technologies, services and software in health while making adherence more plausible as all possible players can be engaged in standards setting. Open content and access provides an avenue for better sharing of knowledge and resources which in turn may be used to boost research in open source software and open standards as well as in health, as a whole. Taken together, these three aspects provide complementary means in building health infrastructure. What all of these have in common is that they go back to the basics of the scientific method in promoting sharing of knowledge as a potent force to further make knowledge grow. It then supports the growth of the information-intensive medical field.

Today, the sustainability of this open architecture becomes more promising. The greater number of players that are attracted in the field provide a network effect—that with increasing numbers of players come greater benefits because more people are able to contribute to knowledge. More and more models to ensure financial and technical sustainability of open source operations are also being proven effective. The challenge of today is to continue to build on the inherent advantages of this open paradigm and to learn from the lessons of its practice to be able to aid in addressing the issues of achieving quality, equity, affordability, appropriateness and accessibility in healthcare.

Appendix—Open Source Software in Health

Hospital Management Information System/ EMR

World VistA (http://www.worldvista.org/)
Programming Language: GT.M.

This is the open source version of VistA, the US-based HIMS that is one of the most comprehensive systems. It's implemented using GT.M., an open source version of MUMPS, which was used in VistA. VistA is in the Public Domain but has proprietary applications that work with it.

Care2x (http://care2x.org/)
Database: SQL-based, XML-based
Programming Language: Java, Javascript, PHP, Perl, PL/SQL
Platforms: OS Independent

It is an web-based integrated hospital information system released in a mature version with a GNU GPL and GNU LGPL license. It is composed of a central data server, health exchange protocol, practice management and hospital information system.

Hospital OS (www.hospital-os.com/en/)

Hospital OS is a free, open source hospital information system used by 50 hospitals in Thailand. Its development is supported by the Thailand Research Fund. It includes registry, scheduling, pharmacy, billing, emergency room, inpatient, diagnosis, ordering, and lab modules.

Electronic Medical Record
OpenMRS (http://openmrs.org)
Programming Language: Java
Database: MySQL

It is an open source electronic medical records system, the development of which is led by the Regenstrief Institute and Partners in health.

Clinical Practice Management
OSCAR (http://www.oscarmcmaster.org/)

OSCAR Canada is a comprehensive suit of FOSS built on Java/Tomcat/MySQL running on the Linux as well as other platforms. It is used in some parts of Canada as well as in Brazil.

CAISI (http://sourceforge.net/projects/caisi)
Programming Language: Java, JSP
Database: JDBC, MySQL, PostgreSQL
Platforms: All BSD platforms(FreeBSD,NetBSD,OpenBSD,Apple Max OS X),
All POSIX platforms (Linux, BSD, UNIX-like operating systems)
This system is based on OSCAR. It offers more features to provide holistic healthcare for homeless people.

OpenEMR (*http://www.oemr.org/* | http://sourceforge.net/projects/openemr/)
Programming Language: PHP
Platforms: Linux, Mac OS X, Free BSD, Windows

Open EMR is free, open source software that has been registered in the public domain since 2002 and presently is already in a production level development. The application includes practice management, electronic medical records, prescription writing and billing applications.

CottageMed (http://www.cottagemed.org/)
Database: Filemaker
Platforms: Mac OS X, PC, Linux

Cottage Med is an open source practice management software being run with a proprietary database, Filemaker. It is being developed by community physicians and is being used already in US and developing nations. Its features include patient billing, scheduling, patient tracking, automated prescription writing, imaging storage and data mining for epidemiology. It also has wireless and PDA support.

PCDOM PrimaCare (*http://pcdom.org.my/*)
Programming Language: PHP
Databse: PostgreSQL

PrimaCare is an open source electronic health records and clinical management system designed for clinics. It presently has modules on system administration, clinic management, financial management, patient management, prescription, billing, schedule, asset and supplies management and medical resources. It is looking into the development of a Generic Engine for Modules (GEM) software to aid in developing modules by providing databases, business logics, user interfaces, and report templates.

MirrorMed (*http://www.mirrormed.org/*)
It is a free and open source web-based practice management system and electronic health record that shares code with FreeMED and OpenEHR. It is a LAMP (Linux, Apache, MySQL) application with a GPL license.

ClearHealth (http://www.clear-health.com | http://freshmeat.net/projects/clearhealth/)
Programming Language: PHP
It is an open source web-based practice management software with a GNU GPL license and that shares code with FreeMed and OpenEMR. It includes scheduling, billing—under the FreeB system, EMR, HIPAA security and accounts receivable. It also has customizable modules for document storage, customizable reporting/forms, lab results and prescription management. Training and migration services are offered by Uversa, Inc.

FreeMed (*http://www.freemed.org* | http://sourceforge.net/projects/freemed/)
Database: SQL-based, MySQL
Programming Language: JavaScript, PERL, PHP
FreeMed is open source web-based practice management and electronic records system with LGPL GNU license. It is already on a production stable release and is maintained mainly by 15 developers. It is supported by the FreeMed Software Foundation, a non-profit corporation promoting the development and acceptance of FreeMed and other GPL and LGPL licenses by contracting grants for their development.

GNUMED (http://gnumed.org)
GnuMed is a python based comprehensive system which is part of the Debian-Med. It has been maintained for several years and is used by doctors in many countries.

Public Health/Epidemiology/Humanitarian
NetEpi (http://netepi.org)
Based on EpiInfo, the widely used epidemiology software from the CDC.

CHITS—Community Health Information Tracking System (*http://chits.mudfish.info*)

Sahana—Disaster Management System—(http://www.sahana.lk/)

EpiSPIDER (Semantic Processing and Integration of Distributed Electronic Resources)
(http://epispider.org | https://developer.berlios.de/projects/epispider/)
Platforms: Windows, Linux
Programming Language: PHP, Javascript

Epispider is an open source web-based software with a GNU General Public License that integrates emerging infectious disease information from the mailing list Program for Monitoring Emerging Diseases (ProMED), a global mailing list reporting on infectious and toxic agents, and Really Simple Syndication (RSS) health news feeds like those from the World Health Organization and Reuters. Natural language processing is done to extract locations from these feeds. Subsequently, these locations are geocoded and presented using Google and Yahoo maps API.

Medical Research
OpenClinica (http://openclinica.org)

The leading open source clinical research application is OpenClinica. It has an LGPL open source license and is commercially supported by Akaza Research which has been created with the goal of promoting shared tools, repositories, and open standards for public research.[52]

Open Infrastructure for Outcomes (http://www.txoutcome.org)

Open Infrastructure for Outcomes (OIO) system enables clinicians, researchers, and other non-programmers to create and maintain flexible and portable patient/research records. Data sets can be exported as XML, Microsoft Excel, SPSS, SAS and other statistical software usable formats.

R Statistics (http://www.r-project.org)
Platforms: UNIX platforms, Windows and MacOS

R is a language and environment for statistical computing and graphics with functions for graphical display, data manipulation and calculation.

Weft QDA—qualitative research tool (http://www.pressure.to/qda)
Platforms: Windows and Linux
    It is free qualitative analysis software application.

TINA—medical image research (http://tina-vision.net/)
Programming Language: C

It is an open source environment for image analysis research. It includes handling of image, image feature, and geometrical data, statistical and numerical analysis, and GUI development. It also has high level analysis techniques (3D Object location, 2D object recognition, temporal-stereo depth estimation) and medical image analysis like MR tissue segmentation and blood flow analysis.

Openbravo—Project Management Software (http://www.openbravo.com)

It is a web-based, open source ERP (enterprise management system).

FreeMind—Mind mapping software (http://freemind.sourceforge.net/wiki/index.php/MainPage)
Programming Language: Java

It is free, open source software with a GPL license. It has many uses including being a workplace for Internet research.

iPath—(http://ipath.sourceforge.net)
Programming Language: PHP

It is an open source platform for telemedicine applications such as consultations, case discussions, and virtual staff meetings. It was originally developed at the University of Basel. Ipath also has a Care2x integration.

Medical Imaging
OsiriX—DICOM viewer for MacOSX (http://www.osirix-viewer.com/)

Medical image processing software for DICOM images rendered by medical equipment like MRI, CT, PET. It is used by more than 20, 000 users worldwide and is fully compliant with DICOM standards.

CD Medics PACS web (http://cdmedicpacsweb.sourceforge.net)
Programming Language: PERL
Database: MySQL 5
Platform: All POSIX, Linux, Mac OS

CD Medics PACS is an open source web-based PACS that is based on ctn or dcm4chee and dcmtk released in a production/stable version with a GNU GPL.

dcm4che (http://www.dcm4che.org)
Programming Language: Java
Database: Jboss

Dcm4che is a collection of open source applications and utilities for healthcare. It includes DICOM storage and DICOM Query/Retrieve to handle DICOM objects. Its WADO and RID components enable web access of the archived content. Dcm4che also incluudes HL7 and IHE services.

OpenSourcePACS Project—(http://www.mii.ucla.edu/index.php/ MainSite:OpenSourcePacsHome)

Open Source PACS is a free, open source image referral, registering, routing and viewing system developed by the UCLA Medical Imaging Informatics. In addition to conventional PACS functions, it integrates wet read functions. It is implemented through DICOM Presentation State and Structured Reporting standards. With it, a primary care physician can order imaging and specify questions that have to be answered with the help of the imaging. Patient's imaging is obtained at the imaging center and the viewer reads the imaging and records annotation which are sent back to the primary care physician.

AMIDE—(http://amide.sourceforge.net)
Programming Language: C
Platforms: Linux, Windows, Mac OS X

It is a free tool for viewing, analyzing and registering of large amounts of anatomical and functional volumetric imaging medical data sets released in a production/stable version under a GPL license. It is able to import many DICOM files, save studies in XML data and create fly through movies as MPEG1,

The Visualization Toolkit (VTK) (http://public.kitware.com/VTK)—
Programming Language: C++ class library, Tcl/Tk, Java, Python
Platforms: Unix-based systems, Windows, Mac OSX Jaguar
It is open source software system for 3D computer graphics, image processing, and visualization.

Raynux (http://www.rad.unipd.it/progetti/raynux/rayUK.php3)
Database: Interbase

Free and open source radiologic software laboratory.

Appendix—Federal Standards

On March 21, 2003, the Departments of Health and Human Services, Defense, and Veterans Affairs announced the first set of uniform standards for the electronic exchange of clinical health information to be adopted across the federal government.[53]

The standards all federal agencies will adopt are:

- Health Level 7 (HL7)[54] messaging standards to ensure that each federal agency can share information that will improve coordinated care for patients such as entries of orders, scheduling appointments and tests and better coordination of the admittance, discharge and transfer of patients.
- National Council on Prescription Drug Programs (NCDCP)[55] standards for ordering drugs from retail pharmacies to standardize information between healthcare providers and the pharmacies. These standards already have been adopted under the Health Insurance Portability and Accountability Act (HIPAA)[56] of 1996, and ensures that parts of the three federal departments that aren't covered by HIPAA will also use the same standards.
- The Institute of Electrical and Electronics Engineers[57] 1073 (IEEE1073) series of standards that allow for healthcare providers to plug medical devices into information and computer systems that allow healthcare providers to monitor information from an ICU or through telehealth services on Indian reservations, and in other circumstances.
- Digital Imaging Communications in Medicine (DICOM)[58] [59] standards that enable images and associated diagnostic information to be retrieved and transferred from various manufacturers' devices as well as medical staff workstations.
- Laboratory Logical Observation Identifier Name Codes (LOINC)[60] to standardize the electronic exchange of clinical laboratory results.

Standards Announced on May 6, 2004:

On May 6, 2004, the Departments of Health and Human Services, Defense, and Veterans Affairs announced the adoption of 15 additional standards agreed to by the CHI initiative to allow for electronic exchange of clinical information across the federal government. The 15 new standards build on the existing set of five standards adopted by HHS in March 2003. The new standards agreed to by federal agencies will be used as agencies develop and implement new information technology systems.

The specific new standards are:

- Health Level 7[61] (HL7) vocabulary standards for demographic information, units of measure, immunizations, and clinical encounters, and HL7's Clinical Document Architecture standard for text based reports. (Five standards)
- The College of American Pathologists Systematized Nomenclature of Medicine Clinical Terms[62] (SNOMED CT) for laboratory result contents, non-laboratory interventions and procedures, anatomy, diagnosis and problems, and nursing. HHS is making SNOMED-CT available for use in the U.S. at no charge to users. (Five standards)
- Laboratory Logical Observation Identifier Name Codes[63] (LOINC) to standardize the electronic exchange of laboratory test orders and drug label section headers. (One standard.)
- The Health Insurance Portability and Accountability Act (HIPAA)[64] transactions and code sets for electronic exchange of health related information to perform billing or administrative functions. These are the same standards now required under HIPAA for health plans, healthcare clearinghouses and those healthcare providers who engage in certain electronic transactions. (One standard.)
- A set of federal terminologies related to medications, including the Food and Drug Administration's names and codes for ingredients, manufactured dosage forms, drug products and medication packages, the National Library of Medicine's RxNORM[65] for describing clinical drugs, and the Veterans Administration's National Drug File Reference Terminology (NDF-RT)[66] for specific drug classifications. (One standard.)
- The Human Gene Nomenclature (HUGN)[67] for exchanging information regarding the role of genes in biomedical research in the federal health sector. (One standard.)
- The Environmental Protection Agency's Substance Registry System[68] for non-medicinal chemicals of importance to healthcare. (One standard.)

Standards Announced 2006:

During 2006, the Departments of Health and Human Services, Defense, and Veterans Affairs announced the adoption of 3 additional standards agreed to by the CHI initiative to allow for electronic exchange of clinical information across the federal government. The 3 new standards build on the existing set of standards adopted by HHS in 2003 and 2004. The new standards agreed to by federal agencies will be used as agencies develop and implement new information technology systems.

- Digital Imaging Communications in Medicine (DICOM) standards to enable the exchange of multimedia information
- Health Level 7 (HL7), SNOMED, the FDA SRS and EPA SRS UNII Codes and RXNORM for the exchange of allergy information
- Health Level 7 (HL7), International Classification of Functioning and Disability (ICF) and related CHI endorsed vocabularies for the exchange of Clinical Assessments and Disability and Functional Status[69]

Appendix—Standards development

Project Initiation

A new standard begins its development at project initiation, when a project is defined and gains approval. The task of developing the standard is then delegated to a technical committee or subcommittee within the organization. Committees are generally composed of volunteers who represent the industry, government, and other stakeholders.

Comments and Review

Committee members create a draft standard through regular meetings and online/ email discussions, and distribute completed sections to the entire group for review and comments. If a subcommittee is developing the standard, a draft will then be presented to the full committee for review and comments. The subcommittee will address these comments, and redistribute the revised draft to the committee for final approval. This process can go through several iterations before a draft is finalized and ready to be approved.

Balloting

Once approval has been received, the draft standard is ready to go to ballot. When a standard goes to ballot, all members of the development organization are able to vote on it. These votes are classified as affirmative, negative, or abstention, and can be accompanied by comments. In order to pass, a balloted standard must win a certain majority of affirmative votes (usually two-thirds).

Draft Standard for Trial Use

If, however, there are no substantive changes, the standard is approved as a Draft Standard for Trial Use (DSTU) available for use by the industry.

From ANSI Approval to Implementation

Once a standard is approved by ANSI as a national standard, its implementation is neither immediate nor even guaranteed—it must first gain traction in the marketplace. For this to occur vendors must first choose to incorporate the standard into new systems as they are designed, and providers then have to either purchase these new systems or upgrade their existing ones.

Because such conversions have a total cost of ownership that can be significantly more than their initial direct costs, and will considerably impact organizational processes and systems, neither vendors nor physicians will commit to such an undertaking without substantial evidence of long-term value.

OMG Adoption process

If we take the OMG, their adoption process is as follows, as copied from their web site[70] :

OMG adopts specifications by explicit vote on a technology-by-technology basis.

The specifications selected each satisfy the architectural vision of MDA. OMG bases its decisions on both business and technical considerations. Once a specification adoption is finalized by OMG, it is made available for use by both OMG members and non-members alike.

Request for Proposals (RFP) are issued by a Technology Committee (TC), typically upon the recommendation of a Task Force (TF) and duly endorsed by the Architecture Board (AB).

Steps in the Adoption Process

A Task Force, its parent Technology Committee, the AB and the Board of Directors participate in a collaborative process, which typically takes the following form:

Development and Issuance of RFP

RFPs are drafted by one or more OMG members who are interested in the adoption of a standard in some specific area. The draft RFP is presented to an appropriate TF, based on its subject area, for approval and recommendation to issue. The TF and the AB provide guidance to the drafters of the RFP. When the TF and the AB are satisfied that the RFP is appropriate and ready for issuance, the TF recommends issuance to its parent TC, and the AB endorses the recommendation. The TC then acts on the recommendation and issues the RFP.

Letter of Intent (LOI)

A Letter of Intent (LOI) must be submitted to the OMG signed by an officer of the member organization, which intends to respond to the RFP, confirming the organization's willingness to comply with OMG's terms and conditions, and commercial availability requirements. (See section 4.3 for more information.). In o rder to respond to an RFP the respondent must be a member of the TC that issued the RFP.

Voter Registration

Interested OMG members, other than Trial, Press and Analyst members may participate in specification selection votes in the TF for an RFP. They may need to register to do so, if so stated in the RFP. Registration ends on a specified date, 6 or more weeks after the announcement of the registration period. The registration closure date is typically around the time of initial submissions. Member organizations that have submitted an LOI are automatically registered to vote. Initial Submissions Initial Submissions are due by a specified deadline.

Submitters normally present their proposals at the first meeting of the TF after the deadline. Initial Submissions are expected to be complete enough to provide insight on the technical directions and content of the proposals.

Revision Phase

During this time submitters have the opportunity to revise their Sub missions, if they so choose.

Revised Submissions

Revised Submissions are due by a specified deadline. Submitters again normally present their proposals at the next meeting of the TF after the deadline. (Note that there may be more than one Revised Submission deadline. The decision to extend this deadline is made by the registered voters for that RFP.)

Selection Votes

When the registered voters for the RFP believe that they sufficiently understand the relative merits of the Revised Submissions, a selection vote is taken. The result of this selection vote is a recommendation for adoption to the TC. The AB reviews the proposal for MDA compliance and technical merit. An endorsement from the AB moves the voting process into the issuing Technology Committee. An eight-week voting period ensues in which the TC votes to recommend adoption to the OMG Board of Directors (BoD). The final vote, the vote to adopt, is taken by the BoD and is based on technical merit as well as business qualifications. The resulting draft standard is called the Adopted Specification.

Business Committee Questionnaire

The submitting members whose proposal is recommended for adoption need to submit their response to the BoD Business Committee Questionnaire [BCQ] detailing how they plan to make use of and/or make the resulting standard available in products. If no organization commits to make use of the standard, then the BoD will typically not act on the recommendation to adopt the standard. So it is very important to fulfill this requirement.

Finalization

A Finalization Task Force (FTF) is chartered by the TC that issued the RFP, to prepare an adopted submission for publishing as a formal, publicly available specification. Its responsibility includes production of one or more prototype implementations and fixing any problems that are discovered in the process. This ensures that the final available standard is actually implementable and has no show-stopping bugs. Upon completion of its activity the FTF recommends adoption of the resulting draft standard called the Available Specification.

The FTF must also provide evidence of the existence of one or more prototype implementations. The parent TC acts on the recommendation and recommends adoption to the BoD. OMG Technical Editors produce the Formal Published Specification document based on this Available Specification.

Revision

A Revision Task Force (RTF) is normally chartered by a TC, after the FTF completes its work, to manage issues filed against the Available Specification by implementers and users. The output of the RTF is a revised specification reflecting minor technical changes.

Goals of the evaluation

The primary goals of the TF evaluation are to:

- *Provide a fair and open process*
- *Facilitate critical review of the submissions by members of OMG*
- *Provide feedback to submitters enabling them to address concerns in their revised submissions*
- *Build consensus on acceptable solutions*
- *Enable voting members to make an informed selection decision*

Submitters are expected to actively contribute to the evaluation process.

Appendix—Open Standards in Health

Open Healthcare Framework (OHF) Project (*http://www.eclipse.org/ohf*)

This project is forwarded to improve interoperability between applications and systems within and across healthcare organizations. It will be implement extensible frameworks and tools for implementations of key health informatics standards based component and support the objectives of many government health departments to encourage the use of interoperable open source infrastructure to lower integration barriers. This framework, components and tools of this project are then to be used by vendors and integrators in applications and gateways in health infrastructures.

ehealth Standardization Coordination Group (World Health Organization) (*http://www.who.int/ehscg/en*)

EHSCG is a group that is involved in the exchange of information on the technical areas of e-health standardization. It strives to identify areas where further standardization is needed and it offers guidance for implementations and case studies. It fuels activities to increase awareness of existing standards and looks into appropriate development paths for health profiles of existing standards to provide functional sets for key health applications.

Health Level Seven (*http://www.hl7.org*)

HL7 is a healthcare Standards Development Organization(SDO), which is American National Standards Institute(ANSI)-accredited. It is particularly involved in creating approaches, standards, guidelines, methodologies and related services for interoperability of data on clinical patient care and the management, delivery, and evaluation of health services.

Clinical Data Interchange Standards Consortium (*http://www.cdisc.org*)

CDISC is an open multidisciplinary, non-profit organization that has established global industry standards in electronic acquisition, exchange, submissiono and archiving of clinical trials data and metadata for medical and biopharmaceutical product development. It is working towards developing and supporting global, interoperable, platform-independent data standards to support research in healthcare.

OpenECG (*http://www.OpenECG.net*)

This project's goal is to promote the consistent use of format and communication standards for computerized electrocardiograms. It further aims to shape development of similar standards for stress ECG, Holter ECG, and real-time monitoring. To be able to do this, information days, workshops and a programming contest are planned. It will also serve to consolidate expertise, assist integration, and support correct implementations. The project involves healthcare authorities, cardiologists, integrators, engineers, standardization bodies, manufacturers, and the public.

OpenEHR (*http://www.openehr.org*)

OpenEHRis an international nonprofit foundation that is geared towards making the interoperable, life-long electronic health record. Its goals are to promote and publish formal specifications for representing and communicating electronic health records, EHR information architectures, models and data dictionaries. It also aims to validate EHR architectures through comprehensive implementation and clinical evaluation while maintaining open source reference implementations and collaboration with other groups working with health information systems.

OASIS (http://www.oasis-open.org/committees/tc_home.php?wg_abbrev=ihc)

OASIS is a nonprofit consortium international consortium that works towards the advancement and adoption of open standards. OASIS standards are pre-approved by an OASIS Committee and subsequently subject under public scrutiny. Then, the standards must be implemented by at least three organizations. The final step is the ratification by the consortium. One of the committees is the OASIS International Health Continuum TC that aims to promote the adoption of OASIS standards in healthcare across already established vertical standards and beyond regional and international interests. Such promotion can include implementation-oriented projects that involve companies to demonstrate the use of these standards. It is to provide an avenue for Healthcare companies to raise their concerns and needs with respect to XML and Web Services based standards. It also aims to provide a mechanism for the documentation of best practices in relation to the adoption of OASIS standards internationally.

OpenEMPI (http://www.openempi.org)

OpenEMPI strives to build an open community that works on development and critical evaluation of open source solutions for use as a community or enterprise Master Patient Index (MPI). Its goals are:

- to articulate an accessible framework for the development of open source MPI solutions in any relevant computing environment
- to discuss and share patient disambiguation, de-duplication and matching algorithms of any type
- contribute towards useful open source MPI implementations for any relevant computing platform
- seek critical appraisal of existing components and recommendations for a standards based approach toward the community development of an MPI. This should include a structured evaluation process, with meta-analyiss, of production open source MPI solutions.

OpenHRE (*http://www.openhre.org*)

Open Source Health Records Exchange Organization aims to build a community that propagates the development, distribution and support of standard Record Locater, Health Record Exchange and Access Control services held as Free/Open Source Software by working with open collaboration among all stakeholders. The end goal is to accelerate implementation of the National Health Information Network(NHIN) by providing Health Stakeholders affordable means to establish the secure and interoperable exchange of health records between existing proprietary and open Electronic Health Records systems by using Free/Open Source Software. It provides support through either the help forum in sourceforge or a fee-based help.

CORBAMed (Common Object Research Broker Architecture Med)

(http://healthcare.omg.org/Roadmap/corbamed_roadmap.htm)

CORBAMed is the health care task force of the Object Management Group (OMG) that is presently composed of about fifty members from vendors, health care providers, payers and end users. It aims to have the OMG technology adoption process to have standardized object-oriented interfaces between healthcare related services and functions. Some of the service areas of interest include : Person Identification Service (PIDS), Clinical Observation Access Service (COAS), Decision Support Services (DSS), Lexicon Query Service (LQS), Security, Record Locator Services, and Encounter Management.

Appendix—Open Content in Health

The Open Directory Project (ODP)—Healthcare *http://dmoz.org/Health/* is the largest, most comprehensive human-edited directory of the Web. It is constructed and maintained by a vast, global community of volunteer editors.

Wikipedia *http://en.wikipedia.org/wiki/Healthcare*
This is the largest online encyclopedia, and is a truly revolutionary concept. It is maintained by a group of dedicated individulas and content is added by the global community of the web.

Open Content Alliance *http://www.opencontentalliance.org/*
The Open Content Alliance (OCA) represents the collaborative efforts of a group of cultural, technology, nonprofit, and governmental organizations from around the world that will help build a permanent archive of multilingual digitized text and multimedia content. The OCA will encourage the greatest possible degree of access to and reuse of collections in the archive, while respecting the content owners and contributors.

Supercourse *http://www.pitt.edu/~super*
A global repository of lectures on public health and prevention targeting educators across the world. Supercourse has a network of over 42500 scientists in 174 countries who are sharing for free a library of over 3232 lectures in 26 languages.

The Public Library of Science *http://www.plos.org/*
The Public Library of Science is a nonprofit organization that publishes freely available open access journals covering all aspects of life science and medicine. PLoS publishes peer-reviewed scientific and medical journals that include original research as well as timely feature articles.

One World South Asia Initiative Section on Health *http://southasia. oneworld.net/article/archive/7525/*
OneWorld is a site that promotes the exchange of ideas with the goal of promoting justice around the globe. It has thousands of text partners, video contributors, and partner radio stations that post multimedia content for free use of the public.

Appendix—Open Access in Health

Free Medical Journals *http://www.freemedicaljournals.com/*
The Free Medical Journals Site was created to promote the free availability of full text medical journals on the Internet.

Pubmedcentral *http://www.pubmedcentral.nih.gov/*
This is the U.S. National Institutes of Health (NIH) free digital archive of biomedical and life sciences journal literature.
Some are called Open Access (OA) articles. In this context, OA means that an article is still protected by copyright but is distributed under a Creative Commons or similar license that generally allows more liberal use than a traditional copyrighted work. The license terms are not identical for all OA articles. Please refer to the license statement in each article for specific terms of use.

Entrez PubMed *http://www.ncbi.nlm.nih.gov/entrez/*
PubMed offers free, online access to the National Institute of Medicine's MEDLINE databases. The site provides access to citations and abstracts from biomedical literature. If a publisher has a web site that offers full-text of its journals, PubMed provides links to that site. While there are some free full-text articles available, many publishers charge a fee for access to full-text. NLM also provides links to biological resources, consumer health information, research tools, and more.

ClinicalTrials.gov *http://clinicaltrials.gov*
The U.S. National Institutes of Health, through its National Library of Medicine, has developed ClinicalTrials.gov to provide patients, family members and members of the public current information about clinical research studies. ClinicalTrials.gov provides easy access to information about the location of clinical trials, their design and purpose, criteria for participation and additional disease and treatment information.

CenterWatch Clinical Trials Listing Service *http://www.centerwatch.com/*
CenterWatch Clinical Trials Listing Service contains trials for many types of diseases. It is searchable by disease categories and geographic area. All of the trials listed are open (enrolling new patients).

Appendix—List of Acronyms

ANSI	American National Standard Institute
APDIP	Asia-Pacific Development Information Programme
DICOM	Digital Imaging and Communications in Medicine
EHR	Electronic Health Record
FOSS	Free Open Source Software
ICD	International Classification of Diseases
ICT	Information Communication Technology
IOSN	International Open Source Network
MDA	Model Driven Architecture
NAHIT	National Aliance for Health Information Technology
OMG	Object Management Group
SDO	Standards Development Organization
PIM	Platform Independent Model
PSM	Platform Specific Model
RFP	Request For Proposals
SDO	Standards Development Organization
SNOMED-CT	Systematized Nomenclature of Medicine—Clinical Terms
UNDP	United Nations Development Program

Endnotes

1   WHO. Preamble to the Constitution of the World Health Organization as adopted by the International Health Conference, New York, 19-22 June 1946, and entered into force on 7 April 1948.

2   World Health Organization. "Fifty-First World Health Assembly: Health-for-all policy for the twenty-first century." May 16, 1998. Available from http://www.nszm.cz/cb21/archiv/material/worldhealthdeclaration.pdf.

3   WHO. Preamble to the Constitution of the World Health Organization as adopted by the International Health Conference, New York, 19-22 June 1946, and entered into force on 7 April 1948.

4   de Savigny, Don, Harun Kasale, Conrad Mbuya, and Graham Reid. *inFocus: Fixing Health Systems*. International Development Research Centre, 2004. Available from http://www.idrc.ca.

5   *New York Times*. "World's Best Medical Care." August 12, 2007.

6   "Thailand Health Profile 2000-2004." Available from http://www.moph.go.th/ops/health_48/chap6.zip.

7   Organisation for Economic Co-operation and Development. "Towards High-Performing Health Systems: Summary Report." 2004.

8   WHO six point agenda http://www.who.int/about/agenda/en/index.html

9   WHO six point agenda http://www.who.int/about/agenda/en/index.html

10   *Wikipedia*. "Health Informatics." http://en.wikipedia.org/wiki/Medical_informatics (accessed October 23, 2007).

11   Fitzmauric JM, Adams K, Eisenberg J. Three Decades of Research on Computer Applications in Healthcare: Medical Informatics Support at the Agency for Healthcare Research and Quality. J Am Med Inform Assoc. 2002; Vol 9 No. 2:144-160.

12   LAMP—http://en.wikipedia.org/wiki/LAMP_(software_bundle)

13   Linux—http://www.linux.org/

14   Apache—http://www.apache.org/

15   MySQL—http://www.mysql.com/

16   PostgreSQL—http://www.postgresql.org

17   PHP—http://www.php.net/

18   Python—http://www.python.org/

19   PERL—http://www.perl.com/

20   Java—http://java.sun.com/

21   Tomcat—http://tomcat.apache.org/

22   Zope—http://www.zope.org

23 NAHIT—http://www.nahit.org/cms/index.php?option=com_content&task =view&id=227&Itemid=201

24 OpenClinica. http://www.openclinica.org

25 BioMail. http://biomail.sourceforge.net/biomail/

26 Kulikowski. 1997. Medical Imaging Informatics: Challenges of Definition and Integration. *The Journal of the American Medical Informatics Association.* 4, no. 3 (June): 252-253. Available from http://www.pubmedcentral.nih.gov/ articlerender.fcgi?tool=pubmed&pubmedid=9147344

27 http://www.hospital-os.com/

28 OSHCA Web Portal - Session #05 - Challenges towards Adoption of FOSS Medical and Health Information Systems in Pakistan. http://www.oshca.org/ Members/twcook/oshca2007_presentations/OSHCA_Challenges_From_ Pakistan_fouadbajwa_final.ppt/view (accessed October 25, 2007).

29 OSHCA Web Portal - Session #05—Challenges towards Adoption of FOSS Medical and Health Information Systems in Pakistan. http:// www.oshca.org/Members/twcook/oshca2007_presentations/OSHCA_ Challenges_From_Pakistan_fouadbajwa_final.ppt/view (accessed October 25, 2007).

30 VistA Implementations in Egypt. Available from http://www.vistasoftware. org/why/sspdfs/VistA_Egypt.doc (accessed October 25, 2007).

31 Valdes. 2006. VistA in Egypt, an Interview with Omar H. El Hattab. *LinuxMedNews*, January 7. Available from: http://www.linuxmednews. com/1136668574 (accessed October 25, 2007).

32 http://www.maximus.com/corporate/pages/adminhealthsyssvs.asp

33 Tolentino H et al., "Linking Primary Care Information Systems and Public Health Vertical Programs in the Philippines: An Open-source Experience," *AMIA 2005 Symposium Proceedings*, 2005.

34 Currion, de Silva, and Van de Walle, 2007. Emergency response information systems: emerging trends and technologies: Open Source software disaster management. *ACM* 50, no. 3: 61-65. http://delivery.acm. org/10.1145/1230000/1226768/p61-currion.html?key1=1226768&key2= 4624415711&coll=&dl=ACM&CFID=15151515&CFTOKEN=6184618 (accessed November 6, 2007).

35 Apikul. 2006. Managing Disasters - Sahana. *UNDP-APDIP International Open Source Network*, September 21. http://www.iosn.net/foss/humanitarian/ projects/sahana/ (accessed November 6, 2007).

36 *National Alliance for Health Information Technology-2005-Adapted from the IEEE definition of interoperability, and legal definitions used by the FCC (47 CFR*

51.3), in statutes regarding copyright protection (17 USC 1201), and e-government services (44 USC 3601)

[37]   ISO/IEC 9126 : Information technology - Software Product Evaluation - Quality characteristics and guidelines for their use - 1991.

[38]   Leape LL, Bates DW, Cullen DJ, Cooper J, Demonaco HJ, Gallivan T, et al. Systems analysis of adverse drug events. ADE Prevention Study Group. JAMA. 1995;274: 35-43.

[39]   Raschke RA, et al.,A computer alert system to prevent injury from adverse drug events: development and evaluation in a community teaching hospital, JAMA,1998,280:1317-20.

[40]   The Value of Computerized Provider Order Entry in Ambulatory Settings, Center for Information Technology Leadership, 2003.

[41]   Evans RS, Pestotnik SL, Classen DC, et al. Preventing adverse drug events in hospitalized patients. *Ann Pharmacother* 1994;28(4):523-7.

[42]   ANSI Standard Development Process http://www.nahit.org/cms/index. php?option=com_docman&task=doc_download&gid=69&Itemid=197

[43]   http://www.whitehouse.gov/news/releases/2004/04/20040427-4.html

[44]   Sfakianakis S, et al. Reflections on the Role of Open Source in Health Information System Interoperability. IMIA Yearbook of Medical Informatics 2007. 2007. pp.50-60

[45]   Kim. 2005. *Clinical Data Standards in Health Care: Five Case Studies.* California Health Care Foundation. Available from http://www.chcf.org/documents/ ihealth/ClinicalDataStandardsInHealthCare.pdf

[46]   Open Content License http://opencontent.org/opl.shtml

[47]   Open Content http://en.wikipedia.org/wiki/Open_content

[48]   Creative Commons Licenses http://en.wikipedia.org/wiki/Creative_ Commons

[49]   Wikipedia http://en.wikipedia.org/wiki/Main_Page

[50]   ODP http://dmoz.org/about.html

[51]   Open Access Overview http://www.earlham.edu/~peters/fos/overview.htm

[52]   OpenClinica. http://www.openclinica.org

[53]   DHHS http://www.hhs.gov/healthit/chiinitiative.html

[54]   HL-7 http://www.hl7.org/

[55]   http://jop.stateaffiliates-asco.org/jopasco/NCDCP/

[56]   http://en.wikipedia.org/wiki/Health_Insurance_Portability_and_ Accountability_Act

[57]   http://www.ieee.org/

[58]   http://medical.nema.org/

59 http://en.wikipedia.org/wiki/Digital_Imaging_and_Communications_in_
    Medicine
60 http://www.regenstrief.org/loinc/
61 http://www.hl7.org/
62 http://www.snomed.org/
63 http://www.regenstrief.org/loinc/
64 http://en.wikipedia.org/wiki/Health_Insurance_Portability_and_
    Accountability_Act
65 http://www.nlm.nih.gov/research/umls/rxnorm/index.html
66 http://www.ncbi.nlm.nih.gov/entrez/query.fcgi?cmd=Retrieve&db=PubMed
    &list_uids=15360858&dopt=Citation
67 http://www.hhs.gov/healthit/documents/chiinitiative/genes_public_full.pdf
68 http://www.epa.gov/srs/
69 http://www.ncbi.nlm.nih.gov/entrez/query.fcgi?cmd=Retrieve&db=PubMed
    &dopt=Abstract&list_uids=12355489
70 http://www.omg.org/

www.ingramcontent.com/pod-product-compliance
Lightning Source LLC
Chambersburg PA
CBHW050340290526
45785CB00006B/2568